Table of

MW01225105

Anti-Cancer Smoothies: An Introduction

A cancer diagnosis can change everything for a lot of people. Suddenly, all the little things you took for granted in your life are reshuffled and prioritized in ways that you never expected. The way you eat is one example of how quickly and completely life can change. Whether you have cancer or you're at risk of cancer because of your family history - the way you eat can have a major impact on your health and your ability to fight or manage your disease. This introduction of anti-cancer smoothies will help you with some alternative meal planning. Depending on the treatment you're pursuing and the medications you'll be prescribed, your doctors may have very specific things that they want you to eat or avoid. That can make meal planning difficult. These smoothies will work well as meals or as snacks and you'll find them tasty as well as healthful.

Cancer Nutrition

It's important to pay attention to nutrition because the cancer is going to drain your body of all the things that make it strong and give it energy. You'll need to replace a lot of the vitamins, nutrients and minerals that certain drugs and treatments deplete. You also want to keep yourself as strong as possible so you're equipped to fight the disease. Your nutritional plan will depend on your cancer, your overall health and your treatment plan. For example, if you're undergoing surgery to have cancer removed, you'll likely be put on a low fiber diet in order to lessen stomach cramping, gas and other digestive and intestinal hazards.

Building your immune system is essential regardless of the cancer you're fighting. When your body is better equipped to fight off diseases and threats, you're in a position of power that can overcome nearly anything. That's why it's important to feed yourself ingredients that include antioxidants for the best possible immune health.

Anti-Cancer Smoothie Ingredients

You may be wondering what your anti-cancer smoothies will contain. It's hard to know what you'll feel like eating and what you won't want to touch.

You might find that your appetite changes dramatically, and things you once loved are now repulsive to you. Don't force yourself to eat things that don't taste right. There are enough smoothie recipes in this book to ensure you're able to find at least a handful that won't make you sick or turn you off. The ingredients you use for your smoothies will be fresh, healthy and excellent at helping you fight your cancer battle.

Think about colorful foods and how great they are for your health. Foods that have rich colors are high in phytonutrients, which are plant compounds that keep you healthy and can inhibit cancer growth. Colorful foods are also rich in minerals and vitamins, which are important nutrients for your body.

Red foods like watermelon, apples, tomatoes, strawberries and raspberries will all help create yummy smoothies that keep you well.

Orange foods are also good for you; tangerines, oranges and carrots as well as squash, sweet potatoes and pumpkin. If you love a seasonally-inspired pumpkin spiced latte as a coffee drink, you'll really enjoy the smoothie you can create to maximize the health benefits of pumpkin while you recover from treatment.

In the **green food** category, your smoothie recipes will include nutrients that really pack a healthy punch. Broccoli, spinach, kale, celery and avocado all carry extra antioxidants that can suppress cancer growth and prevent healthy cells from turning into cancer cells.

There are some other special ingredients that will keep your smoothies tasting good and easy to digest. **Garlic** is a super-food that's well known to the scientific community as well as healthy eaters. Garlic contains a compound called allyl sulfur that slows the growth of cancer cells. A number of studies have shown that increasing your garlic intake can fight off certain types of cancers, particularly stomach cancer, colon cancer and breast cancer. According to the National Cancer Institute, garlic can block the formation of cancer causing agents in your body and it also raises your natural antibacterial capabilities. While you might not immediately think of garlic as an ideal ingredient for a smoothie, when it's mixed with other superb fruits and vegetables, it works.

Spices and herbs will also play a role in cancer fighting smoothies. **Turmeric** is a spice that gives curry powder its bright yellow color. Turmeric contains the curcumin compound, which interferes with the ability of cancer cells to grow and spread. Research has shown that curcumin suppresses multiple types of cancer, including colon, breast and pancreatic cancers. If your stomach and your mouth can't handle curry, which is often where you find spices such as turmeric, you'll be able to get the same nutritional and medicinal benefits by drinking those ingredients in a smoothie.

If you are suffering from stomach upset due to your treatment, **ginger** can help calm your stomach. Ginger is anti-inflammatory, gets rid of nausea, and may slow the growth of malignant cells.

Studies have shown that ingredients in **rosemary** can inhibit the growth of breast cancer cells and ovarian cancer cells. Although testing on humans remains incomplete, rosemary certainly makes your food more tasteful.

Smoothie Logistics

Yes, they'll have tasty and healthy ingredients, but that's not all these smoothies bring to the table. There's also the convenience and the efficiency that's provided by a meal that simply gets prepared in a blender. If you don't have the energy to cook - you don't have to. If you're not feeling up to a meal at dinnertime but you're hungry before bed - make a smoothie. If you need something quick to grab for breakfast that you can take with your pills - a smoothie can be prepared the night before and left to chill in the fridge. While you're fighting off cancer or working hard to prevent it, you need to allow yourself as much rest and peace as possible. Smoothies can help.

This introduction of anti-cancer smoothies is meant to get you ready to experiment. Some of these recipes will seem like they were designed for your specific tastes. Others will seem a little strange. Don't be afraid to experiment and customize. If you like them really cold, throw in extra ice. If your doctor wants you avoiding certain things and incorporating others, you can work around that. These smoothies are meant to be functional as well as fun, so enjoy what you create and let's put these superfoods to work.

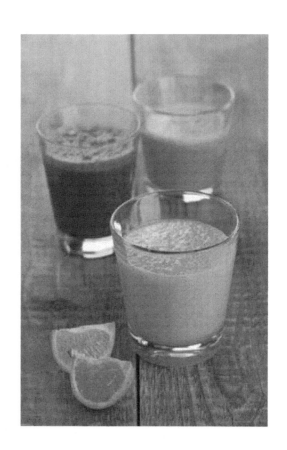

35 Anti-Cancer Smoothies to Try

These anti-cancer smoothies are good for your body and easy to prepare. Check the list of ingredients before you prepare the smoothie and compare it against any lists your medical team has given you. There might be specific foods that you're required to avoid, especially if you are on blood thinners or other medications. With all these options, it's likely you'll find at least a few smoothies that you really enjoy.

1. Super Citrus Smoothie

The citrus fruits in this smoothie provide vitamin C, dietary fiber, beta-carotene and limonoids, and are especially protective against stomach, colon and oral cancers.

1 lime

1 orange

1/2 red grapefruit

1/2 cup plain yogurt

1/2 cup ice

Skin or peel the lime, orange and grapefruit and chop into chunks, removing any remaining skin, fibers and seeds. Place into a blender and add the yogurt and ice.

Blend until smooth. Garnish with a zest from the orange if you appreciate presentation.

2. Bowl of Berries Smoothie

The berries in this smoothie are high in antioxidants, allowing your body to fight off any free radicals roaming around and looking to strengthen cancer cells. Berries can slow the growth rate of malignant cells and prevent tumors.

1/2 cup frozen raspberries

1/2 cup frozen strawberries

1/2 cup frozen blueberries

1/2 cup plain yogurt

1/2 cup cold water

Use frozen berries instead of ice for this smoothie so you don't water down the bursting berry flavors. Toss all the fruits and the yogurt into your blender and give it a splash of cold water. Blend for a few seconds and pour.

3. Apples to Oranges Smoothie

The limonoid compounds in orange and lemon fight oral cancer as well as stomach and colon cancers. Spinach is packed with beta-carotene and lutein that has been shown to be effective against cancer cells. Apples contain antioxidants such as flavonoids, and have been linked with reduced cancer risks.

1 lemon

1 orange

1 apple

1 cup raw spinach

8 ounces of water

Peel, core and remove seeds from the fruits, then chop them roughly. Pour the water into your blender and then add the fruits, followed by the spinach. Blend for 30 seconds.

4. Cranberry Walnut Twist

Cranberries fight off bacteria from your system, giving you a good shot at avoiding some of the illnesses and side effects that come with cancer treatments. Walnuts are full of phytochemical compounds that fight cancer, including polyphenols, flavonoids and omega-3 fats.

1/2 cup frozen cranberries

12 ounces water

4 tablespoons chopped walnuts

1 tablespoon honey

1 orange

Peel the orange and remove seeds. Place it in the blender with the cranberries, water, walnuts and honey. Blend it on high until the walnuts have been ground and the texture is smooth.

5. Pumpkin Pie Smoothie

Pumpkin is a soothing food for cancer patients and can protect against side effects that come with many chemotherapy medications. The beta-carotene that contributes to the pumpkin's autumn color can boost immune systems.

1/2 cup cold canned pumpkin

1 ripe banana

1/2 cup plain yogurt

1/2 cup fresh orange juice

1/2 teaspoon ground ginger

1/4 cup finely chopped walnuts

1/2 cup ice cubes

Combine all the ingredients into your blender and blend on high until everything is combined and smooth.

6. Mad for Mango Smoothie

The avocado in this smoothie will be great for mouths or throats that are tender or sore from side effects to cancer drugs. Avocado is also valuable in fighting cancer by preventing inflammation of cells.

1/2 ripe mango

1/2 ripe avocado

1/4 cup almond milk

1/2 lime, freshly squeezed

1/4 cup ice cubes

Peel the mango and avocado and place them in the blender, covered by the almond milk and ice. Blend on high until smooth, for about 20 seconds. Pour into a glass and drizzle the lime juice on top of the mixture.

7. Blueberry Banana Smoothie

Blueberries contain high levels of antioxidants, keeping your body strong and able to fight off disease.

1 ripe banana

1 cup frozen blueberries

1 cup almond milk

This one is as simple as it gets. Toss the banana and blueberries into the blender with your almond milk and mix it all together.

8. Great Green Smoothie

The green color of this smoothie tells you phytochemicals are at work to booster your immune system and deliver valuable vitamins to your cancer fight. The avocado gives the smoothie a milky texture that's easy to swallow.

1 apple, cored and peeled

1/2 avocado, peeled

1/2 cup apple juice

2 cups raw spinach

8 ounces water

Chop the apple and avocado and toss them in the blender with the apple juice and spinach. Blend together. Add the water slowly in order to achieve the level of consistency you prefer.

9. Rosemary Grape Smoothie

The resveratrol in red grapes is a potent antioxidant that can help treat cancer. Rosemary contains acidic antioxidants that build cancer defenses and help you detox.

2 cups seedless red grapes

1 banana

2 cups baby spinach

Pinch of fresh rosemary

8 ounces water

Blend all of the ingredients together on high for about 20 seconds.

10. Chocolate Avocado Smoothie

Avocado contains antioxidants that can inhibit the development of cancer. If you've lost a lot of your appetite, this smooth chocolate shake will tempt you towards eating and provide a lot of the nutrients you may have lost.

1 cup mashed avocado

1/2 banana

2 tablespoons cocoa powder

1 cup almond milk

Place all of the ingredients in a blender and combine on low for about 30 seconds.

11. You Say Tomato Smoothie

Tomatoes are rich in lycopene, which lowers your risk of cancer. Full of beta-carotene and vitamin C, carrots are good for your immune system.

2 raw carrots, chopped

2 medium tomatoes, chopped

Pinch of salt

Pinch of fresh ground pepper

2 tablespoons freshly squeezed lemon juice

1/2 cup ice

Place the ice in the blender and add the carrots and tomatoes. Blend for five seconds. Add the salt and pepper and blend until the ice is crushed and the vegetables are combined.

12. Coconut-Kale Smoothie

The kale and spinach in this smoothie contain beta-carotene and lutein that are effective against cancer cells.

1/2 red grapefruit

2 cups chopped kale

1 plum, peeled and chopped

1 banana

1 cup raw spinach

8 ounces coconut milk

Pour the milk and fruits into your blender, then cover with the vegetables. Blend on high for 30 seconds.

13. Frozen Cabbage Smoothie

Cabbage is high in antioxidants and anti-inflammatory compounds that can help prevent cancer.

3 cups shredded red cabbage, frozen

1 cup frozen blueberries

1 banana

1 cup almond milk

1/2 cup ice

Break up the frozen cabbage and put it in the blender with the other ingredients. Puree until smooth.

14. Nutty Blackberry Smoothie

Studies suggest that almond consumption may lead to a lower cancer risk, thanks to the nutrients that help preserve a disease-free physical environment. In addition, blueberries and blackberries pack a powerful antioxidant punch.

1 cup blueberries

1 cup blackberries

1 cup almond milk

1/2 cup ice

1/4 cup sliced almonds

1/4 cup walnuts

Chop the walnuts as finely as you can and add them with the other ingredients in a blender. Puree until smooth.

15. The Salad Smoothie

The veggies in this smoothie bring antioxidants and phytochemicals to your diet, upping your ability to fight off cancer cells and stop their spread.

2 cups almond milk

1/4 cup chopped broccoli

1/4 cup chopped cauliflower

1 cup kale

1 medium carrot

1 banana

Pour milk into the blender and add the banana. Cover with the remaining vegetables and blend on high for 20 seconds.

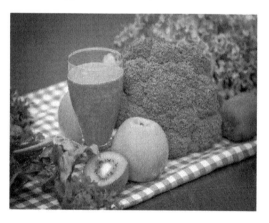

16. Pretty Pear Smoothie

The mild fruits in this smoothie will taste good to sore mouths and rattled digestive systems. Flaxseed can change the way estrogen is metabolized, which is particularly helpful in fighting breast cancer. However, if you have ER+ (estrogen receptor positive) breast cancer, consult your doctor before consuming flaxseed.

1 pear, peeled and cored

2 cups chopped cantaloupe

1 banana

3 tablespoons flaxseed

8 ounces water

Grind the flaxseed as finely as possible and add to the blender with the other ingredients. Puree on high for 15 seconds.

17. Garlic-Almond Smoothie

Garlic is a superfood that contains a compound called allyl sulfur, which slows the growth of cancer cells.

3 cloves of garlic, grated

2 cups almond milk

1 teaspoon apple cider vinegar

1 tablespoon extra virgin olive oil

Sea salt

White pepper

Combine the garlic, milk, oil and vinegar in a blender or mini-chopper and combine. Pour into a glass and sprinkle with salt and pepper.

18. Banana Bread Smoothie

Finding the energy to bake a loaf of comfort food is hard when you're recovering from cancer. This smoothie simplifies the process and provides you with all the cancer fighting ingredients found in walnuts and raisins.

1/2 banana

1/4 cup raisins

3 tablespoons walnuts, chopped

1/2 cup coconut water

1/2 cup almond milk

1 cup ice

Combine all the ingredients in a blender and combine on high speed until smooth.

19. PB&J Smoothie

Peanut butter will give you a protein boost, which is essential for recovery when undergoing cancer treatment. You'll also get the antioxidant benefits of blueberries and the phytonutrients in kale.

6 ounces vanilla yogurt

1/2 cup frozen blueberries

1/2 banana

1/2 cup almond milk

2 cups kale

1 tablespoon peanut butter

1 cup ice cubes

Combine the almond milk, yogurt and fruit in the blender and mix. Add peanut butter, kale and ice. Blend until smooth.

20. Garlic Cucumber Smoothie

Avocado has plenty of cancer fighting properties, but garlic is the real winner in this smoothie. It contains allyl sulfur, which can destroy cancer cells.

2 cloves of garlic, shaved

1/2 cup chopped avocado

1/2 cup cucumber

1 cup chopped green apple

5 mint leaves

1/2 cup water

Fill your blender with all the ingredients and puree until blended and smooth.

21. Celery Zucchini Smoothie

Celery contains the anti-cancer compound apigenin that has been shown to be effective at killing various types of cancer cells.

1 rib celery, chopped

1 tablespoon lime juice

1 banana

1/4 cup zucchini

1/2 bunch of parsley

1 cup water

1/2 cup ice

Place ingredients in a blender and combine on low for 10 seconds. Increase the power to high for the remaining 10 seconds.

22. Green Tea Smoothie

This is a sweet, soothing smoothie perfect for anyone recovering from cancer treatments that upset your stomach. The catechins in green tea are powerful antioxidants and have been shown to reduce tumors in many studies.

1 cup brewed green tea

3 tablespoons fresh lemon juice

1 apple, cored and peeled

1 peach, skinned and chopped

2 tablespoons plain yogurt

1 cup ice cubes

Blend the ingredients until the fruits and ice are pureed and smooth.

23. Ginger on Ice Smoothie

Ginger is anti-inflammatory, gets rid of nausea, and may slow the growth of malignant cells. The strawberries in this smoothie also provide antioxidants healthy for your whole body.

1 tablespoon grated ginger

2 cups almond milk

2 cups strawberries

2 cups raw spinach

1 banana

Blend spinach and almond milk for 15 seconds and then add the remaining ingredients and blend until smooth.

24. Tropical Smoothie

This smoothie provides a strong tropical taste, even if you've had trouble making peace with your taste buds while getting treatment. The compounds in ginger will also help with pain reduction if your treatments leave you hurting.

1 cup fresh chopped pineapple

1/2 cup plain yogurt

1 cup pineapple juice

1/8 teaspoon ground cinnamon

1 tablespoon fresh ginger, minced

1/2 cup ice cubes

Blend all the ingredients for about 30 seconds or until smooth.

25. Mango-Turmeric Swirl

Turmeric has been shown to protect against cancer, making this a great preventative smoothie. Even in patients who already have cancer, scientists have shown that the curcumin compound in turmeric can suppress colon, breast and pancreatic cancers.

1 cup mango

1 banana

2 cups almond milk

1/2 teaspoon turmeric powder

1/2 teaspoon cinnamon

Place all ingredients in a blender and combine on high for at least 30 seconds.

26. Turmeric Watermelon Smoothie

Turmeric, ginger and orange combine to provide the body with a number of defenses against free radicals and cancer cells.

2 cups watermelon, seeded and chopped

1 orange, peeled

1 teaspoon ginger, minced

1 teaspoon turmeric powder

½ cup ice

Blend the ingredients for around 30 seconds.

27. Grapefruit Rosemary Smoothie

If your treatments have left you constipated, this smoothie will help you with regularity. Rosemary is also good for boosting your immune system.

1/2 grapefruit

2 cups raw spinach

1 orange

2 teaspoons chopped fresh rosemary

1 cup watermelon

1 cup ice

1 cup water

Blend the ice with the spinach for 10 seconds and then add the remaining ingredients and combine until smooth.

28. Cranberry Green Tea Smoothie

This is a fresh, tasty smoothie recipe for anyone craving something sweet but lacking an appetite for foods that are filling. The berries are rich in antioxidants, supporting your cancer fight and the green tea will help you detox while building your immune system.

1/2 cup frozen cranberries

1/2 cup frozen raspberries

1/2 cup frozen blackberries

1 banana

2 cups brewed green tea

Cool the green tea after it has been brewed and combine in blender with all the other ingredients. Pulse or puree for at least 30 seconds.

29. Carrot Broccoli Soy Milk

Full of beta-carotene and vitamin C, carrots are good for your immune system. Broccoli contains antioxidants such as indol-3-carbinol, glucosinolates and crambene, which have been associated with lower cancer risks.

1 cup carrots, chopped

1/2 cup frozen broccoli, chopped

1 cup green tea, chilled

1 cup soy milk

Honey to taste

Blend all ingredients together, adding a bit more green tea if the mixture is too thick.

30. What's Up Doc Smoothie

This colorful smoothie looks as healthy as it tastes with all the flavonoids combining to battle cancer cells.

2 carrots

1 cup frozen strawberries

1 cup coconut water

1/2 cup ice cubes

Blend these simple ingredients for 20-30 seconds.

31. Lemon Lime Smoothie

This is a great detox recipe. With the citrus and berries, you'll be able to feel some strength returning and you'll get some vitamins your body needs to replenish itself.

1 lemon, peeled and chopped

1 lime, peeled and chopped

1 cup water

1 cup kale

1 banana

1/2 cup frozen blueberries

Remove stems from the kale and combine all ingredients in a blender.

32. Best Breakfast Smoothie

This smoothie will get you moving on your less energetic days. The carrots will help defend your healthy cells against unhealthy ones and the citrus will keep your system clean, removing toxins that are there to cause trouble.

1 tangerine or clementine, peeled

1/2 grapefruit, peeled

1 banana

1 piece fresh ginger, peeled and minced

1/4 cup shredded carrot

1 cup water

Chop the fruit pieces and combine the ingredients in a blender until smooth.

33. Fruit Salad Smoothie

This smoothie contains all the cancer fighting ingredients such as berries and spinach for their antioxidants and folate. However, the over-ripe banana comes with benefits of its own. The riper the banana, the greater number of antioxidants unleashed in your bloodstream, keeping you stronger.

1 over-ripe banana

1/2 cup frozen blueberries

1/2 cup frozen raspberries

1 cup baby spinach leaves

1 cup almond milk

Put all ingredients in a blender and combine until smooth.

34. Superfoods Smoothie

This savory smoothie will supply you with the super-nutrients that come from veggies. The combination of garlic, spinach and tomatoes will have you better prepared to recover from treatment and fight any potential cancer growth.

2 tomatoes, chopped

1/2 cup red bell pepper

1 cup raw spinach

1/2 avocado

1 clove garlic, minced

2 cups water

Combine the vegetables and cover with water, then blend on high for 30 seconds.

35. Cherry on the Cake Smoothie

Cherries have a number of compounds that prevent cancer and they are excellent for maintaining blood health. They are also great for treating muscle pain, which might be a side effect to the chemotherapy you're receiving.

1 ripe peach, skinned and chopped

1 cup of fresh cherries, pitted

1 cup almond milk

2 limes, juiced

1 cup ice cubes

1 cup spinach

Add all the ingredients in a blender and puree until combined. Taste and adjust with more lime or cherries, depending on preference. If cherries aren't in season, use frozen.

Made in the USA
Las Vegas, NV
14 December 2021

37863566R00016